INCREASES THE
FOCUS WITH THE
ADHD

Increases The Focus With The ADHD

Getting the Most Out of Life with Attention Deficit Disorder

CLIFFORD

Amplitudo LTD

Copyright

Contents

.

Introduction

Introduction

Congratulations on purchasing *ADHD Workbook for Adults,* and thank you for doing so.

In this book, you will find every detail that you need to know about ADHD and then learn the techniques with the help of which you can make your life easier. There are strategies that will help you identify ADHD in a person. Finding out that you have ADHD is one of the first steps towards recovering from the problem. The earlier you identify the disorder, the sooner you will get the treatment, and the faster you will be able to bring your life back on track.

Some of the most common symptoms of ADHD include disorganization, impulsivity, distractibility, and so on, and you are going to learn about all of these symptoms in detail in this book. One of the most common results of having ADHD is that both your personal and professional life is severely hampered. In the case of adults, they often cruise along with life, and eventually, they arrive at a stage when everything seems to be going wrong and falling apart. That is when they are diagnosed with ADHD.

Most people don't understand how frustrating ADHD can be. It is not only contradictory but also confusing. When people have to spend their day-to-day lives with this condition, it easily gets overwhelming. When you go to a specialist for diagnosis, they will ask you a lot of questions, and they will also provide you with a checklist of symptoms that you can go through. Medication alone is never enough to help you cope with the symptoms. You always need more, and by more, I mean that you need to take the help of therapy.

Most of us think that ADHD means a kid who is bouncing on the couch and running wildly around the house. But is that the only type of ADHD that you need to be aware of? No, because ADHD can happen to adults too, and that is not how it looks. In fact, there are several adults with ADHD who are not hyperactive, but they have other symptoms. Some people believe that ADHD is one of the most over-diagnosed conditions, but whether that is true or not, you have to understand that the implications on the life of the person are immense. They cannot keep up with their personal relationships, and they forget about stuff very easily. They make impulsive decisions and might go on a shopping spree all of a sudden just because they feel like it, or they might shift between jobs every month. But more often than not, these people are not particularly happy about the decisions they are taking and so, they regret it later. Their patterns and actions are mostly very self-destructive, and they easily fall into the clutches of depression ad addiction. The effort and struggle that has to be given by an ADHD individual are way more than anyone else who is doing the same thing.

We are not only going to break several myths surrounding ADHD, but we are also going to learn about several tactics that can help you cope with your symptoms and lead a more organized life. I know that maintaining a healthy routine can be your biggest nightmare when you have ADHD but trust me, with the proven strategies mentioned here, you are going to learn a lot of self-control and make a lot of improvement with routines.

I am sure that your doctor is going to suggest some medications for this, but that will not be enough. So, in order to get your priorities straight and getting things organized, you will need the help of a therapist. Whenever it comes to making a choice that needs to be made after considerable thought, it's best if you take a time out and then negotiate. If there are any negative feelings inside you, then they have to be removed by someone you trust in order to be able to make your recovery faster. You need this help, even more, when you think that you have not been able to keep up with the expectations of others.

Another thing to keep in mind is that just because someone is energetic and always enthusiastic about stuff, you cannot predict them to have ADHD. You will always find people who are not the quiet type, and they cannot seem to focus their mind on any one thing. So, they keep changing their focus from time to time. But that doesn't make them a patient of ADHD. In this book, you will learn many such facts about ADHD that are not that well-known among people, and that is what creates so much confusion. I am sure that all of you must have come across family members and friends who were all ready to give you advice on what ADHD is and how it can be cured. But most of them are unknown to what ADHD really is. So, before taking any advice from others, I suggest you read this book and consult a specialist for proper diagnosis.

I would also like to give you a small piece of advice here – don't try to finish this book in a rush. I know that most of you would want to finish it in a week. I know that you are also going to feel a sense of accomplishment once you finish this book, but if you want to truly get something out of this, then you need to learn the strategies by heart. And for that, you need to give this some time. It would help if you blocked time in your calendar with the intention of actually doing some work on your problem while reading this book. You have to remind yourself why you are doing this – it is because you want to. If you want change – a change that is going to stay – then you also need to put in the effort. Remind yourself that you deserve, and that is why you have undertaken this journey. And soon, you will see that with these skills under your belt, navigating through life has become so much easier.

There is no end to the number of books on this subject that you will get in the market, but I am thankful that you chose this one. I have tried my best to explain every detail in the most concise manner possible, and so I hope you enjoy it!

Chapter I

Chapter 1: Understanding ADHD

Chapter 1: Understanding ADHD

ADHD is a very common disorder. More than 10 million cases of ADHD are recorded in India per year. Here we will discuss the disorder in detail about the cause of this disorder, types, diagnosis, challenges faced by people suffering from this disorder, etc.

What Is ADHD?

The full form of this acronym is Attention-Deficit Hyperactivity Disorder. Out of all the people in the U.S, approximately 4.4% of the adult population is affected by this disorder which is mainly neurological in origin. It is more likely to occur to men than to women. 5.4 percent of men are diagnosed with ADHD, whereas 3.2 percent of women are diagnosed with ADHD. It is a disorder that causes a deficiency of attention and causes heightened levels of impulsive and hyperactive behaviors. Patients who have ADHD have low persistence, face difficulty in focusing on a particular thing, and are disorganized. They are always restless and find extreme difficulty in being calm. They often tend to make impulsive decisions because of the hyperactivity, which may end up proving to be harmful to them.

Earlier, ADHD was considered to be just a childhood condition, but now it is accepted to be an adulthood condition as well. The rates of persistence of ADHD vary from 6 percent to 30 percent. The persistence rates can be even higher, too.

Studies have shown that in the last decade, there is a hike in the rate of ADHD diagnosis among adults in the U.S. (Winston Chung, 2019)

Why Does ADHD Happen?

Though the exact causes of ADHD are still unknown, there are certain factors that definitely play a part in the development of this disorder. Let us see some of those factors.

- *Hereditary:* ADHD can be inherited. If your parent suffers from this disorder, you have a risk of inheriting the same. Certain genetic characteristics pass down through the generation. You have a more than 50 percent chance of developing this disorder if your parent has it, and you have more than 3o percent chance of developing this disorder if your older sibling has it. However, the inheritance of ADHD is way more complex, so it is not just because of a single genetic fault.

- *Pregnancy Problems:* ADHD may also develop from certain pregnancy-related problems. A child who is born premature, or is born slightly underweight, has a higher risk of developing this disorder. A child whose mother has had difficult pregnancies earlier is also prone to develop this disorder. The frontal lobe of your brain is responsible for controlling emotions and impulses. So, children having head injuries in this region are at a greater risk of developing this disorder. Pregnant women who drink alcohol or smoke are at a higher risk of giving birth to a child having ADHD. Getting exposed to pesticides, PCBs, or leads, while pregnancy may also increase the chance of the baby developing ADHD.

- *Brain Functions:* After birth, if a child develops some infectious disorder that may affect the brain tissues, like encephalitis or meningitis, then that may affect the working ways of sending signals. This may also induce symptoms of ADHD. Sugar and certain food additives are often considered to induce ADHD. However, researches show that ADHD has got nothing to do with dietary factors.

Chemicals present in the brain, also known as neurotransmitters, work differently in adults and children having ADHD. Even the working ways of the nerve pathways tend to differ. Certain areas of the brain of children having ADHD are smaller or less active than those children who don't have this disorder. The neurotransmitter dopamine also plays a significant role. It is linked to learning, attention, mood, sleep, and movement.

Researches have shown differences in brain activities in people with ADHD and without ADHD. The exact significance is still not clear.

- *Other Factors:* Few groups of people are believed to be at a higher risk of developing ADHD like people who were born premature, i.e., before the thirty-seventh week of pregnancy. People with epilepsy are also prone to develop ADHD. People with brain damage also tend to develop ADHD. This damage can occur either in the mother's womb or can also occur because of a serious injury in the head later in life.

Types of ADHD

ADHD is characterized by hyperactivity, impulsivity, and inattention. Most of the people who don't have ADHD also experience a certain degree of impulsive or inattentive behavior, but people with ADHD experience severe hyperactivity-impulsiveness and inattentiveness. There are three types of ADHD, and each type of ADHD is linked to one or more characteristics. They are as follows:

- *Predominantly Inattentive ADHD*: People suffering from this type of ADHD mostly have symptoms of inattention. Their impulsive nature or hyperactivity is not as much as their inattentiveness. Although, at times, it is possible that they have to struggle with hyperactivity or impulse control, but they are not the main characteristics of predominantly inattentive ADHD. This type of ADHD is more common in girls than in boys.
- *Predominantly Hyperactive-Impulsive ADHD:* People who have predominantly hyperactive-impulsive ADHD have symptoms of impulsivity and hyperactivity more than the symptoms of inattention. Patients having predominantly hyperactive-impulsive ADHD may also be inattentive at times, but that is certainly not the main

characteristic of this disorder. Children suffering from this disorder can cause a lot of dis-
turbance in their school's classroom. They make
learning way more difficult for other students as
well as themselves.
· *Combination ADHD:* If a person has combination
ADHD, then it means their symptoms don't ex-
actly fall under hyperactive-impulsive behavior
or inattention. Instead, they experience a combination of symptoms of both categories.

What Is Adult ADHD?

Being an adult, balancing everything in your life
can be really hectic. If you see that you are constantly
forgetful, disorganized, clumsy, late, and always struggling to meet your responsibilities, then it is possible
that you have ADHD. ADHD, in adults, can cause a lot
of hindrance in both their personal and professional
life. If you were diagnosed with ADHD at childhood,
then it is possible that you carry those symptoms
with you into your adulthood as well. It is also possible that you get diagnosed with ADHD in your adulthood, but while you were a child, you were never
diagnosed with ADHD. It is possible for ADHD to remain undiagnosed in childhood. In earlier days, not
many people were aware of it. Children having the
symptoms of ADHD were mostly termed as trouble-

makers, slackers, dreamers, etc. in the earlier days, which is why chances of ADHD being undiagnosed were very much high at that time.

When you were a child, you may have been able to compensate for those symptoms of ADHD. But when you grow up, it is not that easy to run away from your responsibilities. When you are a grown-up individual, you are expected to run a household, raise a family, pursue a lucrative career, and many more. These responsibilities demand concentration, calmness, and focus, which become very difficult for an ADHD patient to maintain. Even normal people find it difficult to meet up to all these responsibilities. So, for people with ADHD, this is just straight away impossible. The only good thing about this disorder is that it is treatable. With the help of a little creativity, support, and education, you can be able to overcome the symptoms of ADHD. You can even turn some of your biggest weaknesses into your strengths. Being an adult, it is totally possible for you to fight against this disorder and succeed.

The symptoms of this disorder are mostly noticed at a young age. The symptoms become more clear and evident when the child's circumstances happen to change. For example, when they start to go to school, they show clear symptoms of ADHD. Most of the cases are diagnosed when the children are mostly between 6 to 12 years of age. ADHD symptoms generally improve with age, but there are many people who were diagnosed with ADHD in childhood and still continue to face problems when they are adults. Inattentiveness and restlessness do not always mean that you have ADHD, but it's a possibility. So, you should never ignore these things and should get a proper diagnosis.

ADHD Diagnosis in Adults

ADHD diagnosis in adults is way more difficult than that in kids. The main reason is the presence of varied opinions of whether the symptoms list used to diagnose ADHD in children should also be implied while diagnosing ADHD in adults or not. In some situations, an adult exhibiting five or more symptoms of impulsiveness and hyperactivity, or five or more of inattentiveness symptoms, may be diagnosed with ADHD, as listed in the children's ADHD diagnostic criteria. The specialist must ask you questions about the present symptoms. According to the current diagnostic guideline, ADHD in adults can't be confirmed if the symptoms were not present since childhood. In case you find difficulties in remembering the problems you faced as a child, the clinician may ask your parents, closed ones, or even check your old school records to search for any abnormality that you possessed as a child. In order to get diagnosed with ADHD, an adult must have certain effects on different areas of life. If the adult faces problems in difficulty in maintaining relationships with their partner and family, or if he faces difficulty in keeping and making friends, or if he tends to drive his car very roughly, then he is likely to have ADHD. If your problems are recent and not repetitive and old, then you are not going to get diagnosed with ADHD.

Most of the criteria that are used for diagnosing ADHD in adults are mainly focused on the identification of symptoms in children and teens. So, there are higher chances of misdiagnosis in adults. In order to perform a proper diagnosis of ADHD patients, the physicians must know the nuances of ADHD and must also be aware of the overlapping conditions developed in adulthood. Earlier doctors believed that ADHD is a disorder that only children could have, but with time, it is clearly evident that a lot of adults are facing the symptoms of ADHD later in life and are seeking an evaluation in their adulthood. So, the understanding of ADHD diagnosis has improved quite a lot in the last few decades. Most people try to compensate for the symptoms of ADHD in their own way. These undiagnosed ADHD patients often try to fight inattentiveness, impulsiveness, and hyperactivity because they are good problem solvers, creative, and bright. But when they are overwhelmed with continuous increasing challenges and responsibilities, that is when reality kicks in, and they seek medical help. According to a certified adult psychiatrist, the average age of ADHD diagnosis is 39 in his practice.

There is a symptom guide to diagnose ADHD in children, but there is no such guide or manual to diagnose ADHD in adults. The only way of successful diagnosis of ADHD in adults is to run a thorough clinical interview to obtain a detailed medical history. It is imperative that the patient goes to a clinician who is particularly specialized in ADHD. This is to make sure that the clinician will take out time to gather all the required information from you in order to diagnose ADHD in adulthood. The clinical interview may also incorporate neurophysiological testing in order to obtain greater insight into the subject's weaknesses and strengths. This will help to identify any comorbid or co-existing conditions.

Most of the physicians miss out on the differential diagnosis. ADHD symptoms often are the results of different mental health issues like a mood disorder or anxiety. The clinician must have a thorough understanding of the comorbid conditions. The emotional sensitivity resulting from ADHD may also appear as mere anxiety or a mood disorder. It is the duty of the clinician to understand how these symptoms can mimic each other and at what point they differ; otherwise, you will just end up wasting energy, time, and money. A clinician who is trained in just one of these conditions may end up making the wrong diagnosis.

So, the clinician must have proper knowledge of ADHD and everything associated with it in order to perform a successful diagnosis of his or her patients. In order to find a good clinician, it is advised that you go to a directory who will guide you about whom you should pursue. Physicians who have no experience of performing mental health diagnoses must refer their patients to a psychologist or psychiatrist having relevant experience of diagnosing ADHD patients.

What Challenges Are Faced By Adults Who Have ADHD?

Adult ADHD has a massive impact on one's life. If it remains ineffectively treated, untreated, or undiagnosed, it can have adverse effects on the quality of life led by a person and psychological well-being.

- *Career Challenges:* ADHD symptoms like forgetfulness, procrastination, poor concentration, and poor time management may make maintaining a healthy life at the workplace and school very much difficult. Many studies have shown that people having ADHD suffers tremendously in their school life and workplace (Aparajita B. Kuriyan, 2012). Studies have shown that people suffering from ADHD who did not receive proper treatment at childhood faces extreme difficulty in maintaining and gaining employment compared to other people (Anne Halmøy, 2009). They feel a constant sense of underachievement and faces difficulty in following corporate rules, following a 9 to 5 routine, and maintaining deadlines. Another big problem is finances. People having ADHD are prone to have difficulties in financial management, as well. They struggle with due debt, late fees, lost paperwork, unpaid bills, etc. because of impulsive spending.

· *Relationship Problems:* Symptoms of ADHD like impulsivity, inefficiency to follow tasks, low frustration tolerance, and poor listening skills tend to have a detrimental impact on social connections, familial relationships, friendships, and romantic relationships (Ylva Ginsberg, 2014). You may feel tired because of the constant nagging of your loved ones for you to put yourself together. People close to you may feel hurt because of your insensitivity and irresponsibility. The effects of ADHD may lead to loss of confidence, disappointment, hopelessness, frustration, and embarrassment. You can get a feeling as if you can never get a hold of your life and live up to your fullest potential, leaving you with low self-esteem. You tend to hurt your loved one's expectations, ending up hurting them as well as yourself for not being able to meet their expectations.

· *Criminal Tendencies:* Certain researches have linked adult ADHD to rule-breaking, criminality, and other safety and legal issues, which includes a heightened chance of getting into car accidents as compared to other people without ADHD (Zheng Chang, 2017). Certain studies also show that individuals exhibiting ADHD symptoms are more likely to get engaged in various criminal activities compared to other people. A recent study showed that 26 percent of prisoners have adult ADHD (Stéphanie Baggio, 2018).

It is seen that men who had childhood ADHD are 2 to 3 times more likely to be incarcerated, convicted, or arrested in their adulthood compared to those who don't have ADHD. The impulsivity that lies within the people suffering from ADHD impairs their ability to control emotions, behavior, and thoughts. Their self-regulating capability is also damaged. A study showed that there is a link between criminal behavior and impaired self-control (Alexander T. Vazsonyi, 2017).

Children suffering from ODD (Oppositional Defiant Disorder) portray a very disobedient, hostile, defiant, and negative behavior towards the authorities and parents. They often show resentful, vindictive, and angry behavior. They grow up and gradually tend to incline towards various criminal activities. 25 to 75 percent of people having ADHD also have ODD.

· *Substance Abuse Tendencies:* Substance abuse

and adult ADHD are strongly linked. Substance Use Disorder or SUD is very common in patients with ADHD than those who have not been diagnosed with this disorder. In fact, it is two times more likely to happen to ADHD patients. Many adults suffering from ADHD and having a SUD report uses drugs and alcohol to manage ADHD symptoms and self-medicate.

· *Comorbid Disorder:* 60 to 70 percent of people suffering from adult ADHD have a comorbid disorder. According to a study on adult ADHD, about 15 percent of them were found to have a substance abuse disorder diagnosis, 50 percent of them were found to have anxiety disorder diagnosis, and 40 percent of them were diagnosed with a mood disorder (Benjamín Piñeiro-Dieguez, 2016).

· *Health Issues:* ADHD symptoms can also contribute to a wide range of health problems like chronic tension, stress, substance abuse, compulsive eating, etc. People suffering from ADHD often tend to forget to take vital medicines, skip doctor's appointments, ignore medical instructions, neglect vital checkups, and thus are more likely to get themselves into trouble.

If you suffer from ADHD, then that might not be the only health issue you have. ADHD often brings other health issues along with it. Adults suffering from ADHD may have health issues due to alcohol and drugs, sleep problems, depression, etc.

- *Depression:* ADHD is very much likely to make you feel frustrated and sad at times. Clinical depression is very much different than just being sad. It is way more severe and causes the day to day problems in social activities, relationships, school, work, etc. 70 percent of the people who have ADHD get treated for depression at some point in their life.
- *Sleep Problems:* Problems with sleep cycles are very common in people who have ADHD. Even kids with ADHD find it difficult to obtain enough rest. People with ADHD are two to three times more likely to have sleep problems than those who don't have ADHD.
- *Serious Behavioral Problems:* People with ADHD often develop ODD (Oppositional Defiant Disorder). In this, people tend to resentment and anger without any proper reason. They often have a tendency to blame others for their own bad behavior. They purposely annoy people and tend to break the rules and argue with everyone.

Another behavioral disorder noticed in people with ADHD is CD (Conduct Disorder). ODD often turns into CD and becomes more severe. Forty-five percent of teens who have ADHD tend to develop CD later in their life, and 25 percent of children suffering from

ADHD also develop CD later in their life. People with CD tend to skip school, steal, destroy properties, and shows extreme aggressive behavior towards animals and people.

Chapter II

Chapter 2: Common Myths About ADHD

Chapter 2: Common Myths About ADHD

Misconceptions and myths can be found in every minute portion of life, and thus ADHD is no different. However, when myths and misconceptions start forming deeper roots in society, it can make the whole situation turn into some major problem. People start believing them, and the ultimate result is that you won't be able to differentiate between true and false. That is the primary reason why misconceptions and myths regarding any kind of disease can result in serious harm. So, it is essential to debunk such myths and just see the problem in the real light. Also, myths and misconceptions can sometimes make the treatment procedure quite tiresome. We will debunk some of the primary myths about ADHD in this chapter so that you do not end up misunderstanding your child.

ADHD Cannot Be Regarded As a Real Disorder

ADHD has always been recognized as a serious disorder by most medical professionals, psychological and psychiatric experts, and organizations and associations in the United States. Some of the major organizations are APA or American Psychiatric Association, NIH or National Institute of Health, along with the Center for Disease Control and Prevention. One of the primary factors that actually contribute to myths or misunderstandings about the status of ADHD is that there is a lack of any proper test that can truly identify the disorder. Just like other serious medical conditions, a medical expert or a doctor cannot just confirm the diagnosis of ADHD with the help of imaging and laboratory test. Indeed there is no proper test for the diagnosis of ADHD; there are certain specific and clear criteria that require to be met for the diagnosis. Mental health professionals and doctors can put into use these criteria, along with detailed history and information regarding the concerned person's behaviors, to provide a reliable diagnosis.

Another important factor is that the symptoms of ADHD are not always defined clearly. ADHD exists on a proper sequence of behaviors. All of us experience some sort of problems regarding focusing and attention at times. However, for a person who is suffering from ADHD, all these symptoms might turn out to be severe enough that they can easily hamper their daily functioning. ADHD symptoms might also resemble some other conditions. Undiagnosed or pre-existing medical problems need to be recognized before the diagnosis of ADHD.

ADHD Is Often Over-Diagnosed

The evidence regarding this is kind of mixed. According to annual data, there is an increase in the diagnosis of ADHD in children in the U.S. But the reports also state that the rates of other serious conditions, like anxiety, depression, and autism, have also shown an increase. Talking about ADHD in specific, various studies have demonstrated that the condition might get under-diagnosed in certain cases where the overall symptoms are much less noticeable. A prominent example gathered from the pieces of evidence shows that ADHD might manifest in a different way in female children. While female children suffering from ADHD have fewer chances of showing any kind of hyperactive symptoms, they might still have some impairment of significant kind with focus and mental tasks. A wide range of studies has suggested that female children are less likely to get diagnosed and also receive any kind of treatment related to ADHD than male children.

Some other studies suggest that ADHD is most of the time over-diagnosed, however, particularly in boys. Increased rates of ADHD in male children might be partly because of the stereotypes regarding male behavior; for instance, boys tend to act out physically. Boys might also be more likely to show disruptive and ADHD symptoms, which directly enhances the chances that teachers, parents, and also doctors will notice all their behaviors. It has been found that ethnic, socioeconomic, and racial factors also play some role in the disparity in the treatment and diagnosis of ADHD. In accordance to a study from the year 2016, white children were most likely to be diagnosed with ADHD and also receive treatment for the same. Although the researchers find these findings to imply over-diagnosis, they suggest that under-treatment and under-diagnosis of Latino and African American children with ADHD could be a more specific interpretation of the gathered data.

Another research proposed that ADHD in adults is also over-diagnosed. It is often suggested that adults might get diagnosed with the symptoms of ADHD because of the medicalization of their typical personality variations and life experiences. In some of the cases, other types of learning disabilities or mental health conditions are often misdiagnosed as the symptoms of ADHD. The primary risk involved with the over-diagnosis of ADHD is unnecessary treatment along with stimulant medication. Although the related drugs can work as an effective treatment for ADHD, when provided to someone who does not require them, they might be misused.

ADHD Can Only Be Found In Children

The ADHD symptoms require to be present by the age mark of seven years to properly meet the criteria of diagnosis. However, there are people who often remain undiagnosed until they reach adulthood. It not at all uncommon for some parents to get diagnosed with ADHD along with their children at the same point in time. As any adult starts learning in detail about the actual condition, they might start recognizing the traits of ADHD along with the related behaviors in themselves. While thinking about their childhood, they might just realize that the struggles they faced at school were most probably the result of problems related to attention that went untreated or unnoticed. For children and parents, proper diagnosis at any point might seem like a relief. Getting the ability to put the symptoms under some kind of names while also knowing that there are ways to properly manage them might be reassuring.

A lot of children, who get diagnosed with the symptoms of ADHD, might continue to showcase the symptoms even as teens and adults. However, the overall nature of the symptoms might change as they grow. For instance, the hyperactive nature of behaviors that are common in kids has the tendency to reduce with age. However, distractibility, inattention, and restlessness might persist into their adulthood. ADHD in adults, which is managed poorly, might often result in chronic problems in relationships and at work. Untreated and undiagnosed ADHD can also be linked with substance misuse, depression, and anxiety.

ADHD Is the Result of Bad Parenting

Parents of ADHD children might often worry that they are the ones to be blamed for the behaviors of their children. However, the overall condition is not caused by bad parenting strictly. Any child, no matter they are suffering from the symptoms of ADHD or not, can get affected adversely by critical and punitive parenting or a chaotic home. All such factors might make the whole situation tougher for the children to cope with the problems of ADHD; however, they are not the primary cause of the condition. With that said, parents might want to consider adapting their style of parenting to support their ADHD child in a better way. It has been found that children suffering from ADHD tend to benefit from consistent and clear consequences and expectations, along with having some predictable nature of routine at their home.

One of the Surest Symptoms of ADHD Is Hyperactivity

The 'attention deficit' portion of the name has resulted in misunderstandings regarding the overall nature of the condition and has also perpetuated various myths regarding the symptoms. In fact, there are various ADHD types that we have already discussed in the previous chapter. Hyperactive behaviors can be found only in the predominantly hyperactive-impulsive type and cannot be found in the predominantly inattentive one. In order to reduce any kind of confusion, ADHD of the predominantly inattentive nature is often referred to as attention-deficit disorder or ADD. Any individual who showcases inattentive symptoms might appear easily distracted and daydreamy. They might also be careless, forgetful, and disorganized. ADHD of this type is overlooked most of the time. It is mainly because it is of a less disruptive nature than the hyperactive one. But the related symptoms can still be dreadful to the one who is experiencing all of them.

While any child suffering from ADHD would not outgrow the disorder typically, sometimes adults report growing out of the behaviors of hyperactive nature that they had in their childhood. In some cases, hyperactivity might get replaced by apathy and restlessness.

People Suffering From ADHD Cannot Focus At All

Provided the name of the condition, it might be really confusing for some people to see someone with ADHD/ADD intently focusing on any activity. It will be more accurate to describe the portion of 'attention-deficit' as difficulty in regulating concentration in place of the ability to pay any attention. Although individuals suffering from ADHD face difficulty organizing, completing, and focusing on tasks, it is not at all uncommon for them to get absorbed in all those activities that they find interest in. In fact, hyperfocus of such a sustained level can indicate when someone has ADHD.

Stimulants Might Result in Addiction and Drug Abuse

There is a major concern that the stimulant medications that are used for treating problems of ADHD can result in substance misuse. But it has been found from researches that ADHD, when left untreated, can easily enhance the risk of a person for the disorder of substance use. Depression or anxiety can also result from untreated ADHD. An individual might misuse illicit and licit drugs in order to medicate their symptoms of ADHD along with any other secondary nature of the psychological condition. It has also been found that all those who receive proper treatment for ADHD come with a lower percentage of substance misuse, along with stimulant medication.

Medication Can Completely Treat ADHD

Medication cannot cure the symptoms of ADHD. However, it can readily help in managing the symptoms when administered under the guidance of mental health professional. ADHD can be regarded as a lifelong and chronic condition. If someone gets prescribed to have ADHD medication during their childhood, they might have to continue consumption of the same as an adult as well. People might just carry on with the same symptoms as adults that they had as children. The symptoms might also lessen or just change with time. Developmental alterations in the brain can explain all such changes partly. However, they might also be the reflection of the ways someone has gained knowledge about coping.

Individuals suffering from ADHD might often develop organizational skills and coping strategies to help them move on with the condition. They can just expand and continue to build up all these skills all throughout the course of their lives. They might also decide to pair the same along with medications.

ADHD Develops When Children Are Lazy

It can be regarded as a proper way of demeaning the actual problem as ADHD is not a result of a lack of motivation or laziness. It is an actual medical problem that needs to be addressed properly. When your child is suffering from the symptoms of ADHD, it is not the case that he/she is not trying to focus on things. In actuality, they are giving their best to do so. However, they cannot end up doing so. In case you are just asking your child to concentrate more and being rude/angry on the, as they are not trying, it is actually worthless. It is similar to getting angry at someone as they cannot see something, while in reality, they are actually blind. Your child's attitude is not the main factor that is trying to affect the child's attentive power. It is only because of some physical differences that exist in their brain for which they cannot do or see things like any other child. Expecting them to perform or behave like the rest of the children when they are not even built in that way is foolish.

In fact, there are cases where people do not even clearly understand the concept of ADHD and blame their children for not focusing on something or behaving a particular way. All of this indirectly worsens the symptoms of the child and also makes him/her feel guilty. When your child is suffering from the problems of ADHD, you will have to develop a huge number of reminders to make them actually do some task. However, that does not indicate that your child is lazy. All it means is that they do not possess the brain structure to dedicate so much effort. Even playing a very easy game of building blocks might turn out to be mentally tiring for a child who is suffering from the symptoms of ADHD. So, it will be better for them if you can just stop judging them or comparing them for staying behind other children.

Myths and misconceptions regarding ADHD might turn out to be harmful at many levels. Myths can make timely diagnosis a difficult job. Understanding and awareness of ADHD can help a lot in combating various kinds of challenges that are faced by the sufferers of the same.

Chapter III

Chapter 3: Diagnosis of ADHD

Chapter 3: Diagnosis of ADHD

Have you not been able to finish any work this week? Do you keep losing your house keys all the time? Are you feeling terribly disorganized in your life? As you know, from Chapter 2, all of these symptoms definitely point to ADHD. But you also have to keep in mind that ADHD is much more than these symptoms alone. So, never jump to any conclusions before you visit a specialist. If you think about the different symptoms of ADHD singularly, you will realize that they are not really that abnormal. Feeling restless or forgetting things is very common. Even if your distractibility has reached chronic levels, it doesn't mean that you have ADHD.

The problematic part is that ADHD cannot be diagnosed through any physical or medical test. If you want to know whether you or your child is suffering from ADHD, you have to visit a specialist or a health professional who performs such a diagnosis. They implement a lot of different psychological tools to predict whether you have ADHD or not. They might ask you about your past problems or even the present ones, and you have to answer them honestly; they might even make a checklist of symptoms for you or prescribe some medical examinations that will help in ruling out certain other causes that might be behind those symptoms.

A proper diagnosis is very important because there are several symptoms like hyperactivity and loss of concentration that not only happen in ADHD but in a whole lot of other problems as well. This is why ADHD can be confused with a lot of other medical problems leading to a wrong diagnosis. It is also confused with certain emotional problems and learning disabilities just because there is an overlap in the symptoms. The problem with the wrong diagnosis is that the affected person will then not receive the treatment they deserve or require to cure their actual problem. So, keep in mind that just because your symptoms match with that of ADHD, it doesn't mean that it is ADHD. A thorough diagnosis aided with a properly researched assessment by a specialist is necessary to conclude it as ADHD.

Factors That Are Looked Into

Like I told you earlier, the specialist might you a set of questions that will help him/her to make a proper diagnosis. Every person displays different symptoms when it comes to ADHD. So, in order to make a proper diagnosis, there are different things that have to be considered by the professional and set the criteria accordingly. You should also promise yourself that you are going to be as honest as you can while answering the questions of the specialist; otherwise, the diagnosis will not be accurate.

In short, if someone has to be diagnosed with ADHD, they will have to show strong symptoms. These symptoms are a combination of inattention, impulsivity, and hyperactivity. They are known as the hallmark symptoms of ADHD. But just to give you an idea, some of the factors that the specialist takes note of are as follows –

· **What is the severity of the symptoms?** – If someone has to be diagnosed, then the symptoms that they are having should be severe enough to hamper their life to a great extent. It applies to both children and adults. If you see people who have already been diagnosed with

ADHD, you will notice that multiple facets of their life have been gravely affected because of ADHD, and this includes their personal relationships, work, and even financial responsibilities.

· **Do the symptoms show themselves at a particular time?** – If you indeed have ADHD, then the symptoms will pop up in multiple settings and not just in one place. You will face symptoms at the workplace, at home, and even when you are out on a date. It is probably not ADHD if you are facing the symptoms at only one place or one time of the day.

· **When was the first time you noticed the symptoms?** – This is another very important thing to take note of in the diagnosis of ADHD. In the case of ADHD, the symptoms generally start appearing the childhood years. In some cases, people get diagnosed later on when they reach adulthood. Also, if you are an adult, then the therapist might help you trace your current symptoms back to the earlier years and help you think whether you faced them even before or not.

· **How long do you have the symptoms?** – This is somewhat related to the previous question, but here is something that you should know – if anyone is to be diagnosed with ADHD, the symptoms should be persisting for at least six months. It is only after that the specialist can rule it as ADHD.

How to Choose a Specialist for ADHD Diagnosis?

If someone has ADHD, whether it is an adult or a child, they are going to face problematic situations every day and so, getting them the right treatment is very important. There are a lot of specialists that you can go to for getting yourself or your kid diagnosed.

- **Primary Care Doctor** – The first option that is open in front of you is your primary care doctor or general practitioner. They will perform basic diagnosis, and depending upon the situation, they might either refer you to some psychiatrist/psychologist, or they can even prescribe medications.
- **Psychiatrist** – A psychiatrist is a highly trained medical professional in the scope of mental health. They are definitely one of the best people to help you with ADHD diagnosis and prescribe the right meds. They can even give you therapy and counseling sessions. If you are seeking a diagnosis for your child, then it is better that you visit a psychiatrist who already has experience working with kids in the past.
- **Psychologist** – When a health professional seeks a degree in psychology, they are referred to as a psychologist. They can offer you with

different types of therapies like behavioral therapy and social skills therapy. They can even assist you in testing your child's IQ and, after that, take the necessary steps to mitigate the symptoms. In a few places, psychologists also have the power to prescribe medications, but in other places, psychologists are not always allowed to prescribe. In that case, they will ask you to visit a doctor who can prescribe meds.

Now, we come to the question – how are we to find a specialist who meets all our criteria and is right for us? This person should be someone you are comfortable with. Sometimes you might not find the right person at once. You will have to make appointments with some of them, visit them, and then decide for yourself whether you like them or not. That is why it is advised that you go to your primary care doctor, get an initial diagnosis, and also ask him/her for a reference. If you know someone who has ADHD, then you can also ask them for a reference. If it's your child who you think has ADHD, then you can also contact the school and ask them for a reference suitable for a child.

Your next step should be to call up your health insurance company. Sometimes these treatments are not covered, and at other times, they are. You can also ask them for names of specialists if the treatment is covered under the package. Once you have narrowed down to the prospective specialists, call them up, ask them for how long they have been practicing, and any other questions that you might have.

Here are some of the things that you can ask –

- What is their usual line of treatment for ADHD?
- Have they worked with children before, and if yes, then for how long?
- How can you make an appointment with the doctor?

Before you find the person who is a perfect fit for you, it is quite natural that you will have to do a bit of hit and trial. The person that you finally choose should be someone who has a welcoming attitude, and you think that you will be comfortable talking to them. If, after a few appointments, you or your child are still struggling with building a bond, then I think it is time that you look for another therapist.

Diagnostic Challenges

As already discussed, there are a lot of challenges related to ADHD diagnosis. The major one being that some people are not diagnosed in their childhood years. The symptoms are not expressed in the same manner in children and adults. The reason behind the complexity of the diagnosis process of ADHD is that it depends on a lot of historical data of the patient, and all this information needs to be accurate. The process of collecting all that data and ensuring that it is correct can be quite challenging and also a tedious task. AHD can develop anytime after the age of 12. And if the person who is going to the specialist is already an adult, then he is going have a lot of trouble remembering things that happened when he was 12 years old.

A multi-source assessment has to be made to make the results concrete. Thus, different sources have to be used. Some of the examples include – history of employment records from school, any interviews that the person might have attended, and so on. So, going through all the available records and looking for diagnostic clues everywhere is how a proper diagnosis is made. The developmental problems are going to become even more commonplace if the person has a family history of consistent ADHD. Any member of the family having ADHD completely changes the game because then the genetic factor is added.

Moreover, if someone does have ADHD, then they do not have the best memory, and thus, their accounts of what happened earlier cannot simply be trusted. When asked, they might say that they are facing problems in some aspect of their life when, in reality, nothing like that is happening there but in some other aspect of their life. So, do not trust anything that the patient has said unless and until you have cross-referenced it with something else. That is why diagnosis is advised to be done in a combination of feedback tests from colleagues, school records, and families.

The society that we live is provided us with a daily amount of stimulation that can lead to the formation of ADHD like symptoms. So, at any particular point in time, there is a lot of things on your plate competing to get your attention. On top of all that, you might also feel stressed because of your personal relationships. If someone lives in a dysfunctional family or works at a chaotic office, then it can not only cause inattention but also cause mood disorder.

The comorbidity rates in the case of ADHD are so high that it often causes a lot of confusion. It causes distraction, and people are no longer sure whether it is ADHD or not. There might be some obvious disorders in a person that is easily diagnosable, but he/she might also have ADHD that is subtle. In such a case, the diagnosis of ADHD is overlooked. Only a very patient diagnostician with an informed approach can rule it as ADHD if they keep an eye on all the other co-existing problems.

Another challenge that is faced is that certain drugs that are used in the treatment of ADHD have a tendency to induce addiction. So, there are people who tend to fake ADHD just because they want to get hold of those drugs. At the same time, this same problem might lead to a denied diagnosis of those who truly have ADHD. So, when someone is making a decision regarding the diagnosis of ADHD, they should be considering both sides of the story.

Here is something else that should be kept in mind – sometimes, patients are overpathologized by the diagnosis. That is not what an ideal situation should be. The ultimate aim of diagnosis is to give the necessary help to the person. The diagnosis should not convince the person that he/she is a failure, or it should not give them an excuse to give up on their lives. The diagnosis should be the first step towards selecting the most effective form of treatment for that person.

Step-By-Step Guide to Diagnosing ADHD

Here I am going to guide you through a step-by-step approach to ADHD diagnosis –

SOCIAL, ACADEMIC, AND EMOTIONAL FUNCTIONING ASSESSMENT

This is the first step in ADHD diagnosis. The different aspects of life are evaluated, and this holds true for both adults and children. Once a detailed assessment report is made, it will be compared to kids who do not have ADHD to see what is abnormal and what is normal.

There will be checklists and questionnaires regarding the behavior of the patient – this is basically a self-report. In case the patient is a child, a 'report by other' is also done, and in that case, the questionnaires and checklists will have to be answered by someone who spends a lot of time with the child. Once all of these reports have been completed, a score is calculated. This score is the point of comparison to find out what is ordinary and what stands out and might be a possible symptom of ADHD. Several standardized rating scales are also used by specialists in order to evaluate the information. One of the most important parts of the comprehensive assessment of a child or adult is the behavioral checklist. But these reports cannot solely diagnose ADHD. They are just a part of the process.

After the behavioral checklists, it is time for the intelligence tests, which are also very crucial. There are some standard tests that are done first, and then once the findings arrive, some special tests might also be done depending on the findings. Tests of daily functioning, achievement tests, and intelligence tests are some of the common tests that are done. These can further include personality tests, memory tests, and symptoms checklists. There are two basic components of intelligence, and these are judged by these tests. These components are – the ability of a person to learn from what happened before and the ability to adapt to new situations. Basically, when these intelligence tests are conducted, the specialists are looking for any inconsistencies in the cognitive and behavioral patterns that are usually present in other disorders. One of the prime requirements of these tests is a consistent level of mental effort, which is something ADHD patients struggle with. The tests require a person to be fast-paced, attentive, and solid memory skills, all of which are not present in ADHD patients. Moreover, in most of these tests, the instructions are not repeated more than once. So, it is because of these tests that the intellectual functioning of a person can be judged.

Next, the achievement tests are usually designed to judge the person's skills in specific subjects. It can be mathematics or even oral language. Sometimes, diagnosing ADHD becomes easier because kids who have ADHD have a specific performance pattern in these tests. That pattern can then be used by experts to make a future diagnosis as well. Scores are usually high when a particular task does not require the person to engage in sustained effort. On the contrary, scores are low when the task requires sustained mental effort and concentration.

As you know that ADHD patients have trouble paying attention, and so, the next test done during the diagnosis are the tests of attention. Even though it might sound like an easy test for you, it is not. There are four different aspects of attention, namely, sustained attention, alternating attention, selective attention, and divided attention. In order to find what the weaknesses and strengths of a patient are, all the aspects of attention are tested.

Once this is done, we move on to the last test that is done in this step – the memory test. Although, apart from the memory test, some other small general tests are also done. The memory test examines not only the patient's long-term memory skills but also short-term memory. The tests measure their distractibility, delayed memory, retrieval from memory, and auditory and visual memory.

CLINICAL INTERVIEWS

The second step in the process of diagnosis is the round of clinical interviews. These interviews are constructed to get information about the patient's educational history, family, and other personal facts. Detailed histories are collected not only from the patient but also from the other close people in his/her life. Everyone might have a different perspective, and once this interview round is over, all the perspectives are arranged in order to form a complete picture.

Some of the information that is asked to the care-givers or parents of the patient are as follows –

- How have the symptoms been progressing ever since they showed themselves?
- When or under what circumstances did the symptoms first appear?
- Under what settings are the patients facing functional difficulties, and how severe are they?
- What impact are the symptoms having on the family and the patient?
- Is the family of the patient capable of giving him/her the care they need at this moment?

Once the initial interviews with the caregiver or the family members are over, the specialists will then talk with the patient. The patient will always have his/her questions about the situation. Listening to their side of the story is equally essential for diagnosis. It can be quite a challenging process, especially if the person is not open to the idea of seeking the help of mental health professionals. The age of the patient is a huge determining factor as far as the perspective is con-cerned. But this step is vital because it will make the patient more open to the idea of treatment, and they will gradually become comfortable with the process.

MEDICAL HISTORY AND PHYSICAL EXAM

Now, no matter what diagnostic assessment we are talking about, it can never be complete without checking what the overall health of the person is. It is even more critical if the person has started showing the symptoms only recently. If the symptoms did not show themselves gradually and were rather sudden, then the cause might not be ADHD in the first place.

The medical history of the patient will be demanded as part of the routine process. So, if the patient has any pre-existing medical conditions like asthma, allergies, epilepsy, and so on, then they have to declare it. The specialist might also ask questions related to the presence of psychiatric illness in the family.

Once all of these processes are complete, the doctor will look through all the conclusive findings and determine whether the patient has ADHD or not.

Chapter 4: A Step-by-Step Guide to Become More Productive With ADHD

Chapter 4: A Step-by-Step Guide to Become More Productive With ADHD

Adults with ADHD often go through days when they feel like they cannot do anything. They cannot think straight, nor can they stay focused on any task—this inability to focus hampers their productivity levels. But the worst part is that this feeling is very often what every day looks like for an ADHD patient. We all know that when it comes to productivity, the most common rules that apply to usual circumstances are prioritize, focus, and delegate. However, these rules cannot be used in the case of an ADHD patient. It is because the ADHD brain works differently.

But no matter how many obstacles stand in your path, it doesn't mean that you cannot be productive. You can definitely learn some strategies that will help you manage your time and stay up to date with work. So, in this chapter, we are going to have a look at some of the most common productivity tips that are extremely useful for ADHD patients and will help you handle every distraction that comes your way.

Step 1 - Don't Try Multitasking

People often think that multitasking is the answer to your problems but trust me, it is not. Multitasking will only complicate things further for an ADHD patient. If you want to get something done, the first and foremost thing is that you need to stay focused. So, for a person who is easily distracted, doing one thing at a time is a big challenge. If that person were to do multiple things at a time, think how hard it is going to be for him/her to stay focused. Every task on that person's list ends up staying incomplete.

You might think that multitasking is going to save time, but it is quite the opposite. When you have to do many things at once, the ADHD brain is not able to work efficiently. The main reason behind this is that there is a constant shift of focus from one task to another, so the brain basically keeps doing back and forth. Every time the brain has to focus on something new, it takes a couple of seconds to readjust. Even if it doesn't seem much to you, these seconds keep adding up, and at the end of the day, multitasking is the reason why you are left with incomplete tasks.

But the problem is, multitasking has become like second nature to most of us. Here are some things that you can do to avoid multitasking –

- Firstly, you have to find out the pairs of activities that you usually tend to multitask. Then, sort them into groups. All tasks that have some kind of familiarity between them can be sorted together in one group. For example, you can watch TV and file your nails at the same time. But you definitely should not answer your emails while watching TV. The idea is to separate the daily tasks which can be grouped together to multitask and save time. But the more complex tasks should be set aside.
- For the tasks that you have pointed out as complex, you need to block time in your planner. This time span will be solely devoted to completing that one single task. When you are spending time doing that one single task, you need to keep your phone away. You can also put

up a board on your door that says 'do not disturb.' If you think that the new project that has been assigned to you is not the typical easy ones and you need extra time to complete it, then let your client know about it.

· Try developing a morning routine. A morning routine might not be directly related to multitasking, but it helps you establish a pattern, and you will do the same things every day in the same order. Moreover, a routine will increase your familiarity with a single task, and the more you do it, the more familiar you will find it. And then, after a certain point of time, that task might become so familiar to you that you can add it to your list of tasks that are multitaskable.

Lastly, I would like to say, no matter what, you should try not to multitask because it has been seen that the more people try to multitask, the more they are late at completing things. This makes them work on the weekends or stay up late every night just to catch up with everything. The result of all this is stress, and you definitely don't want more of that in your life.

Step 2 - Be Realistic

Being realistic is one of the major things to learn in

order to increase your productivity with ADHD. You have to understand that since you have ADHD, your brain is not like that of others. It is different, and the concept of time is also different.

So, when you decide a time frame for your tasks, you need to be quite realistic about it. Keep in mind that every task is going to take much longer than you think it would. So, plan some extra time in your schedules so that you don't have to run at the last minute to cover your deadline. Also, whenever you are planning your tasks and your time frames, include small breaks in between. This will prevent your brain from getting tired, and you will stay energized throughout. Taking breaks in between is all the more important for patients with ADHD; otherwise, your concentration levels will falter.

Thus, you simply have to follow the rule of 'under-promise and over-deliver.' Make it your motto. If you are an optimistic and career-oriented person, you already have an idea in your mind regarding the number of things you can do in a day. But when you promise people around you that you are going to deliver the service within a time period and then fail to deliver it, there is no value in your promise. Moreover, this will also create a constant pressure upon you. So, the trick is to commit less and deliver more. This will not only enhance the satisfaction of the clients but also improve your productivity levels and give you more motivation.

Step 3 – Stop Trying to be Perfect

The need to be perfect at all times is often the biggest hindrance that we have on our paths. And for an ADHD patient, this is all the more true. You have to understand that sometimes it is okay to make mistakes and not do things perfectly. In order to be productive, sometimes you have to allow your laundry to keep stacking in the corner of the room and order takeout. You need to learn to cut yourself some slack from time to time because you are not a machine. Perfectionism is your enemy, and you cannot give in to it. The more you chase perfectionism, the more you will ask yourself whether you are enough. The truth is – 'You are enough.' It doesn't require you to be perfect to be enough. Being perfect is an illusion, and you have to break free.

If you think that you want to be perfect, then you will constantly be chasing something or the other in your life – be it more beauty, wealth, more promotions, or anything. The road of being perfect is always dissatisfying because it will drive you down a track where you will keep wanting for more, and there is no end to that.

Don't depend on others to make you feel worthy

because that is also how perfectionism keeps growing. You will never feel enough if you keep relying on others. It is a deceptive cycle. External validation will inevitably make you feel that you need more to feel enough. So, you need to bring a change to your mindset. Set expectations that are realistic and always put your well-being first. Your perception of the world depends quite largely on how you see it. People are not born with the idea of self-reliance. You have to learn it. The moment you do that, you will realize that you are in more control of the situation than you thought you were. It will not only boost your happiness but also your sense of self-esteem. Accept yourself for the person you are.

Stop telling yourself that you are a failure. This type of negative self-talk is not going to get you anywhere in life. It will not convince you to accept yourself. What you need to do is make yourself believe that you are good just the way you are.

One of the most prominent aspects of striving to be perfect is the need to always get it right. The moment things go a bit off-road, people feel like a failure. But you have to make yourself understand that the fact that you are trying to achieve your goal and putting yourself out there is a huge accomplishment. So, make progress and give a pat on your back because you deserve it.

Step 4 – Prep Your Environment

The next thing to do if you want to be productive is to prep your environment. It will elevate productivity levels by helping you to focus. Whether you are working from home or from your office, your environment plays a significant role in your productivity.

Here are some things that you should keep in mind –

· **Lighting** – The first aspect to take care of is the lighting. If you want to feel inspired to work and churn out more ideas, you'd be amazed to know what a great role lighting plays in it. But even then, people often overlook this factor. You will feel irritated and put a lot of strain on your eyes when your workspace doesn't have sufficient lighting. In fact, it has been found that people become depressed when they work in dark spaces. If you are working from your cubicle at the office and the general lighting is not enough, don't be shy to bring your own light. But if you are working from home, things are in your control. So, allow as much natural light as you can. Open all the windows. If the day is cloudy, make sure you switch on the lights.

· **Table and chair** – Now, let us talk about the type of chair and table that you should use.

When your table and chair are not of the right type, you will often find yourself moving or stretching from time to time. For the best ergonomics, your feet should not be dangling. They should be either resting on the floor or on a footrest. Your eye level should match with that of the top of the monitor. The distance between your eyes and the computer screen should be at least 24-36 inches. In order to avoid or prevent any kind of back pain, the chair posture needs to be a bit reclined. But if you are working in a company, you can't do anything about the chair. What you can do is add some pillows to adjust your back. But if you are having a height problem with the chair, you can ask for a riser. Investing in a good-quality chair is what you should do if you are working from your home.

· **Reduce clutter** – ADHD patients often forget to clean their spaces, but clutter will only hamper your productivity, and you cannot afford to do that. In your office, you obviously do not have control over the clutter generated in the whole area. But you can definitely keep your own workspace clean. Make it a routine to clean your desk every evening before you leave, and every morning when you come. Just set everything in place and start your day fresh. It will help minimize the distraction. When you are working from home, the chances of clutter increase a lot. Everything that is in your house can distract you. If you are someone who stays busy most of the time, then you will need to have a professional cleaner to help you out. But if you want to save money, then you have to fix a day in a week when you will clean everything. Apart from this, set aside fifteen minutes of your time every day to clean your home office.

· **Room temperature** – You might be surprised to know that room temperature does play a role in your productivity. It applies even more to ADHD patients because they tend to get irritated by the slightest things. Your productivity increases with warmer rooms. But in offices, the general temperature that is maintained is 65-68 F, and this is not the ideal range for productivity. Since you cannot control the temperature of your office, you can bring a space heater for your cabin. But if you are at home, you need to adjust the temperature depending on the weather.

· **Room scents** – Your mood is hugely affected by the different scents in your surroundings, and so you should do something about it. If you feel that you have been drifting off quite frequently, then keeping some aromatic substances in your surroundings might help you focus. For example, the smell of cinnamon can help you maintain your focus for longer periods, the smell of citrus helps in lifting up your mood and keeps you awake, the smell of lavender should be used after a long and tiring day at work to help you relax, and the smell of pine keeps you alert. Remember that if you are working in an area where you have others close to you, then you should use scents that are subtle and won't disturb others. But if you are at home, then you can use essential oils or candles.

· **Level of noise** – The level of noise is something that is very often not in our hands to control. The company culture and the size of your team are some of the things affecting the noise. The design of your office also plays a role. But we cannot deny the fact that our concentration levels depend on the noise to a huge extent. If the levels are way above average, then you might find it difficult to concentrate, and your productivity will take a hit. While working from home, people often think that maintaining a quiet space can be attention boosting, but it is quite the opposite. Complete silence is often a distraction in itself. So, you can play some mild sounds that boost your concentration. White noise is a very good example. If you are working from your office or a place that is too noisy, always carry your noise-canceling headphones. They can be a real savior in such situations.

Step 5 – Time Your Tasks

In this step, we are going to learn how you can time your tasks and how beneficial it is when it comes to time management. Timing your tasks can actually give you a better sense of time. And it is also quite simple to do. All you need is to set the alarm on your phone or use a timer. ADHD patients often struggle with procrastination. Timing the tasks will help you deal with it effectively. Fix a particular amount of time for a particular task and then start working. But whatever time you choose, make sure you are not pushing yourself too much. You will know that it is time to start the next task when your timer goes off.

Similarly, when ADHD patients start doing something that they love, they tend to spend the entire day on the task. In order to prevent that, timing the task will let you know that you have already spent a specific amount of time on that task, and now, it is time to move on. It is advisable that you use a timer for every task that you do in the day, be it running errands for home or working on projects at your office.

Timing your tasks will also help you keep track of all those areas where you are less productive, and then, you can work on these areas separately. Every activity that is present on your to-do list for the day should be assigned a specific time span.

Step 6 – Do the Fun Stuff First

I know that many of you believe in doing the difficult things first so that by the time half the day has passed, you are done with the tricky tasks. But in the case of ADHD patients, if the day starts with tasks that pose a lot of resistance, it is easier for them to lose focus. So, it is advised that you do the easier things first. Or, you can start with the things you love doing.

Moreover, when you finish the good things first, it will not take you much time. The sense of accomplishment that you will get on completing those tasks will motivate you to work more and get more things done.

Taking small steps at the beginning of the day will prevent you from getting overwhelmed.

Step 7 – Use Visual Reminders

Visual reminders have often proved to be very helpful for ADHD patients to remember stuff. Moreover, you can be as creative as you want while planning these visual reminders. Decorate your office walls with boards where you can put up your deadlines and personal acronyms to remind you of the tasks that you need to get done. You can also put up rules that you need to follow.

Make sure you put up these reminders and deadlines where it is easy for you to notice them. It will also constantly remind you to use your time productively. You can also take the help of sticky notes to put up reminders on your desk, on your computer screen, or wherever you feel would be easier to notice. You can also set productive screensavers on your computer so that even when you are taking a break, you always have a quote boosting you up.

So, I hope that you follow all these steps mentions here, but the most important thing to keep in mind is that our own negative self-talk is what holds us back. No matter how many tips you follow, if you don't stop automatic negation in your mind, it is only going to put you in a counterproductive path.

Chapter 5: Managing ADHD Behavior Outside the Boundary of School

Chapter 5: Managing ADHD Behavior Outside the Boundary of School

Your child cannot be at home all the time, and there are various other places where he/she will have to go apart from their school. It is your responsibility to teach your ADHD child to properly manage all their behavior in every other place as well. Well, this chapter will be helpful for all those parents who are planning to go on a family trip with their ADHD child.

Traveling By Car

One of the primary things that most ADHD children dread is traveling by car. It might turn out to be a challenge for the parents as well. It is because children who are the victims of the symptoms of ADHD generally prefer to be in their routines only. Their sense of order might get easily hampered by simple out-of-the routine things, such as long rides by car. All of this can result in a phase of tantrums and turmoil. The ultimate result of this is that the family finds it tough to travel anywhere by car anymore. However, in this section, you will come across some simple suggestions that might help you in making your experience of traveling by car with your ADHD child a better one the next time.

· In case you are going somewhere with your child that involves traveling by car, you will have to prepare him/her mentally before few days of going for the trip. You just cannot wake up one morning and tell your child that you will be traveling somewhere that will involve traveling by car for four to five hours or even more than that. You will need to prepare your ADHD child for the alteration of routine along with the scenery that is going to come. If you really want your child to make him/her feel at home even while

traveling, you will have to accept all their suggestions regarding all those things that they
would like to carry with them. You will also have
to explain to your child the motive of the trip or
the destination that you have decided to travel
to. Also, you can tell him/her about the road and
the sceneries that they can enjoy at the time of
travel. In this way, you will get the chance to
prepare your child mentally for the trip.

· Try to maintain at least some portions of their
daily routine as you travel. For instance, try to
wake up your child at the same time as they
do every day. If you just try to wake up your
child one hour before one or two hours of their
daily time, he/she might not be in a good mood.
In fact, the chances of them throwing tantrums
might also be high. So, try to avoid scheduling
all your trips that are way ahead of the daily routine of your child.

· In case the overall time of traveling by car is
quite long, your ADHD child might like to take
a short nap. However, they are used to sleeping
in their bed, and sleeping in the car might seem
odd to them. So, it would be a superb idea if
you can bring their favorite blanket or favorite
stuffed toy in order to make them feel comfort-

able in the car. ADHD children tend to feel se-
cure by the sense of familiarity.

· If he/she starts looking exhausted or tired after
a certain point of time, opt for taking a break
and just stop somewhere. When your child fails
to have enough sleep, the ADHD symptoms
might start worsening. You cannot just let that
happen, specifically when you are traveling. So,
try to encourage your child to take small naps
if you are traveling for a long time or in case
you still have some great amount of distance to
cover.

· Try not to change the determined behavioral
rules. You will have to make him/her realize that
only because they are not at home and traveling
somewhere by car does not provide them a free
pass to do anything they feel like. In case he/
she starts misbehaving, ensure that you remind
them of the related consequences.

· There are several simple things that actually
matter when you have decided to travel with

your ADHD child by car. He/she might just not comply with all that you say or as simple as putting on the seatbelt. In case your child is not at all listening to you, try not to jump to the system of getting them reminded of the consequences right away. In place of doing that, understand why he/she is actually acting grumpy. In order to keep your ADHD child cheerful, you can try to make them a part of the conversation that you are having with other family members.

· You will also need to maintain the social etiquette of your child whenever you are traveling outside. You can opt for giving your child gentle reminders and just follow the process of reminding them of the related consequences in case they keep behaving rudely.

· A very common commotion that ADHD children have at the time of traveling by car is the seating arrangement. Sometimes, children might have some special preferences for their seating. They might even get moody in case they are not permitted to sit in their preferred seat. You will need to teach them how they can share and also maintain a mutual seating arrangement.

· Another common problem that tends to arise on road trips with ADHD children is the part of going to the washroom. In case the trip is long, it is quite a natural thing for you to stop for washroom breaks. At first, your child might want to go to the washroom as you want to go. However, soon after that, they might start throwing tantrums regarding going to the washroom right away. That is the reason why you will have to ensure that your child gets done with their washroom activities right before you leave so that there is no need for them to go to the washroom anytime soon. Even if he/she wants to go to the washroom after some time, make them know that it is tough to locate a toilet on the road. So, they will need to wait for some time depending on the availability of washrooms and the road.

How to Deal With Your Child's Bad Behavior in Public Settings?

Do you always feel tensed and worried regarding the tantrums that you think your ADHD child might throw whenever you go to a public place with him/her? Behavior turns out to be a serious issue with children suffering from the symptoms of ADHD. No matter whatever you ask them to do that they actually do

not want to, he/she might just lash out in an aggressive way at you. Whenever an ADHD child is overpow-
ered with an array of strong emotions that they might
not deal with until and unless they showcase some
form of emotional outburst or act out. However, you
will have to do something regarding their misbehav-
ior right now as otherwise, in case it gets neglected
and gets fostered, after a period of time, your ADHD
child might just develop an oppositional defiant disorder or ODD. Also, according to some reports, ODD has
been found in about 40% of children who are suffering from the symptoms of ADHD.

WHY DOES ADHD CHILDREN ACT OUT?

Right before we delve deeper into the management
of behavioral patterns of ADHD children, you will
have to understand why do they act out in the first
place. Try to think about the history of ADHD of your
child and the ways in which they have been fighting
to deal with the same since childhood. In fact, it has
been found that children suffering from ADHD tend
to get attracted to all those things which they should
just stay away from. For instance, if you ask your child
to behave properly, he/she might just get attracted to
all forms of malicious intent. That is the main reason why, whenever you are out in public with your
ADHD child, and you ask him/her to sit in one place,
they would just run around that place or start speaking loudly. All of this can easily make you feel stressed
in public settings. In fact, it is because of all such situ-

ations that result in negative interactions between the ADHD child and you.

As you keep telling your child from an early stage during their childhood that behavior of this sort is not right and they should stay from them, the child might just start feeling that there must be something wrong with them. So, they just start internalizing all the feelings that they have. At times, they might just act out towards all those people who ask them to stay away from such behaviors or things.

REASONS WHY ADHD CHILDREN THROW TANTRUMS

In the last section, we have discussed in detail the reasons why ADHD children tend to act out. Now, we will discuss the reasons why they opt for throwing tantrums. Children suffering from the symptoms of ADHD usually have to give in a lot of extra effort in getting things done that seem repetitive or boring to them. It indicates that he/she has to deal with a lot of resistance, which makes all their tasks more challenging automatically. In case the task is not permitting them to opt for things that they love or like, for instance, watching TV, they might just decide not to do the task at all. This, in turn, would take the shape of a battleground. These are nothing but strategies of avoidance that your ADHD child tries to opt for. However, for you, they just turn into power struggles quickly, along with being acts of defiance.

When your ADHD child starts throwing tantrums, you might make up your mind to alter the conditions of the overall task so that all of it gets easier for him/her. All of this will make your child feel that they have got the power to throw unnecessary tantrums any time they feel like as you keep reducing conditions for the sake of them.

STRATEGIES TO DEAL WITH TANTRUMS

Let us now discuss the various ways in which you can keep the bad behaviors of your ADHD child under proper control. All forms of disciplinary strategies that are used for other kids might just not work for children who are suffering from the symptoms of ADHD. It is because of one primary reason – you have already developed some form of negative interaction with your child. In fact, if you truly want the strategies to function in the best way for your child, you will have to keep your temper under control. If your ADHD child does not showcase bad behavior every now and then, then raising your voice or just speaking to them firmly might work for bringing them back on track. However, the main problem lies with all those ADHD children who have imbibed it as a habit to misbehave. If you just keep raising your voice or shout at them as you talk, they just think of that to be normal. So, they will just stop paying any form of attention to whatever you do.

Additionally, when you opt for giving too much punishment, the effectiveness of all of that will soon disappear. They will assume that they are living in a world of perpetual punishment, and so it will slowly lose all its meaning. He/she might not just think of it as a big deal when you punish them, and so there will be no effect if they get punished one more time. However, in order to bring your child on track, something can be done on your part.

· When you succeed in introducing a structured routine or lifestyle in the life of your ADHD child, it has been found that he/she might get some sort of benefit from the same. It indicates that you will have to provide them with a proper set of directions or instructions whenever you want your child to do something. You will have to aim towards writing down everything that you are actually expecting from your ADHD child so that they get aware of the same. In case you fail to make your child understand which behaviors are correct and which behaviors are not, how are they going to differentiate between right and wrong?

· There is a very common term that all of you must have heard – scaffolding. In case a child is facing some sort of behavioral problems, then to properly regulate their behavior, they will need a perfect family environment. Also, if you want your ADHD child to learn something great in life, you will have to provide him/her with a proper structure to do so.

· You will need to develop a positive relationship with your ADHD child. The importance of this tends to increase if you want to mend the disruptive behavior of him/her. It is because when there is a bad relationship between the parent and the child, everything seems to be negative. And thus, the disruptive behaviors will just tend to escalate.

· One of the primary reasons why ADHD children showcase bad behaviors is that they are unable to regulate their emotions. So, you will have to work with your child in order to make them more aware of all their emotions. You will also need to teach them the ways in which they can practice self-control. We have already discussed self-control in Chapter 5.

Helping Your ADHD Child in Group Situations

There will be a number of situations where your ADHD child will need to work in collaboration in a group. It might be in their school or even at some party or when they decide to go out and play with other children. However, navigating in this sort of group situation is something that the majority of ADHD children face a problem with. Also, if a proper form of care is not taken, the situation might escalate quite quickly. In the end, the overall group exercise will just leave a negative nature of impact on your ADHD child. Similar to other children, if someone is suffering from the symptoms of ADHD, it does not hamper their desire to make new friends, or be a part of group activities, or even succeed in life. In order to help your child with the same, there are certain things that you will have to do to help him/her.

- Indeed, most of the parents are well aware of the fact that ADHD is a true disorder, and they will have to deal with the same with proper care. However, there are still groups of parents who do not tend to believe in the existence of this disorder. You will have to understand that the symptoms of ADHD in your child are not at all a result of your upbringing. It is nothing more than a disorder in the brain, and it also does not reflect the intelligence of your child. When you try to think that the symptoms of ADHD are not serious at all, you might just start taking all their bad behaviors and tantrums as being willful. All of this can easily make the situation worse.

· You will need to develop a routine before changing the gears. In case you have decided to take things to a higher level in group activities, provide your ADHD child with proper time to prepare for the same.

· To properly deal with all the extra energy that is possessed by your ADHD child, it is your duty to encourage them in various forms of positive opportunities in which they can spend all their energy. As you try to channelize the energy of your ADHD child towards something positive, the chances of them misbehaving or acting out will be less.

· There are some correction strategies that you will have to use as they will help your ADHD child with all their group activities. Try not to criticize anything that he/she does. When your child finally starts taking their steps in the correct direction, you will have to appreciate them in place of just telling them the ways how they can be more perfect. There is no need to push your child in the direction of perfectionism as they are not required to be perfect. All that they need to do is to just continue with all that they are doing.

· At times, you will find that your child is acting out aggressively. However, they do not mean most of the things that they say. It is because their self-control level is low. However, it does not indicate that they will be willing to emotionally hurt you. So, ensure that your reaction to anything is calm. Try not to act out immediately to make them understand by using some form of punishment.

· Try not to be attentive to the negatives. For instance, do not keep telling them all the time what they are not supposed to do. It is because your child might start feeling restrictive. Try to tell them all those things that they should actually do. It will help in the promotion of positive activity in him/her.

· If your ADHD child has been harnessing negative energy, you can just ask him/her to get some simple chores done for you so that all forms of negative energy get out of their body and mind.

· Try to refrain from accusing your ADHD child of anything. You will need to understand and accept the very fact that your child is a slow learner. You will have to provide them with all the time he/she needs. There is no use in pushing them towards something within a fixed timeframe. They will take the time they need, no matter what.

It is a true fact that going outside with your child who is suffering from the symptoms of ADHD is a challenging task. It is mainly because their mood will keep changing all the time during the course of the day. He/she might be excessively happy now and just get sad in the next moment. Also, children suffering from ADHD come with a low level of tolerance. So, they are most likely to get frustrated easily. However, if you start following the steps that we have discussed in this chapter, you can easily learn to navigate slowly through all types of situations.

Chapter VI

Chapter 6: Tips to Make Your Life More Organized

Chapter 6: Tips to Make Your Life More Organized

One of the biggest challenges when a person has ADHD, is to become organized. But it is not something impossible. You can bring structure and discipline to your life if you put in the effort. Always remember that the secret to becoming organized is to follow some simple steps that you can continue doing and having a system that works well for your routine. In this chapter, we are going to have a lot at some simple tips that will help you make your life more organized.

Throw Out What You Don't Need

We all have things in our lives that we keep on accumulating even though we don't need them. And in the case of people with ADHD, these things are even more because they have very poor organizational skills. The more physical clutter you have in your life, the more will be your mental clutter. So, it would be best if you eliminated all those things you don't need from time to time. If you can't figure out where to start, then here are some things that you can throw away –

- **Plastic Grocery Bags** – These things tend to get accumulated in our houses very easily. If you are feeling like going green, just take all the plastic bags that are lying around and visit the nearest recycling center. Then, visit the supermarket and buy some reusable grocery bags. Keep about five of them in your car so that whenever you go somewhere, you always have one in the car. You should buy a bunch more to keep in your house. But in case you are at a store, and you don't have your reusable bags with you, you can always ask for paper bags.
- **Extension Cords** – I know that most of us are guilty of keeping worn out extension cords in our home. But ask yourself whether you really

need so many of them. You can just keep one from each type of cord and throw away the rest.

· **Old Electronics** – Do you hold on to your old gadget even when you have bought a new one? That is how you are giving rise to clutter. You need to get rid of the old one. Or, you can also replace your old one and get a new gadget – this might even save you some money.

· **Extra Bedsheets** – Open your linen closet and see how many bedsheets you have. Every one of us keeps extra bedsheets in case we need them when guests are over. But do you have too many? If so, then you need to discard some of them.

· **Manuals** – In today's when you have everything you need online, why keep accumulating manuals? The first page of the manual might have the warranty card – you can tear it off and throw the rest of the manual away. Even if you need to know something about your device, all you need is the model number, and you will find every information online.

· **Free Samples** – Do you feel good when you get free samples with other products or when you travel? Of course, you do but think about all those times when these free samples just keep accumulating, and we never really use them. So, instead of throwing these samples away, you can donate them to those who really need them.

· **Magazines** – Do you have magazines lying

around in every room? If yes, then you need to make a list of magazines that you really love to read, and anything that is not on that list should be recycled. Also, prioritize the magazines to see whether you still want to continue your subscription to all of them.

Set a fixed day every month when you will go through your belongings and throw out things you don't need. After that, your focus should be on buying things that you absolutely need. If you don't buy unnecessary things, you will not have clutter in the first place.

Maintain a Planner

When you have ADHD, you often tend to forget things, and that creates even more chaos in life. But a simple solution to this problem is maintaining a planner. So, if you have been feeling that there is not enough time in the day for you to do everything, a planner can sort that out for you. You can now keep every errand, every meeting, and every event scheduled so that you don't forget about it. Make sure you keep some time extra on your hands when you note down the event in your calendar. If the meeting is at 2 pm, note down the time as 1:45 pm, so that you have some extra time to give you a cushion.

Once you start maintaining a planner, you will see how your personal and professional life undergoes a huge change. You are going to become so much more productive and no more putting off things for later. If it is included in your planner, you have to do it now. Whatever task we are talking about, a planner will help you stay ahead of things and keep some extra time for you and your family at the end of the day.

Constantly feeling overwhelmed is something very common with ADHD patients, and this leads to an immense amount of stress. But your schedule can be so much less hectic if only you maintain a planner. Every responsibility will be completed seamlessly. You can also use your planner to keep track of what you are eating and whether or not you are doing some regular exercise.

Another important thing to keep in mind is that even when you are maintaining your planner, you need to keep checking it from time to time to ensure that you are not missing out on anything. Make it a habit to note down all your meetings and appointments in the planner. If you don't want to do it manually, you can also use an app for it. Then, you can set timely reminders for everything that is on your planner.

Organize Your Finances

The next step to becoming organized is to have a look at your finances and make sure everything is in order. The forgetfulness that comes with ADHD often makes people overlook their finances, and by the time they realize that it needs work, it is too late. If you don't want that to happen to you, I think you should review your finances every quarter. Mark a particular date in your planner or calendar when you want to review all your financial statements and make sure you do those things on that date. This should be a comprehensive review and must include your retirement accounts, all your bank accounts, and your investment accounts.

If you do not use online banking, then it is high time that you do so now. It is going to make your life so much easier. Writing checks and doing all the work manually is such a hassle. But when you do it online, it becomes way easier. If you think about all the monthly bills that you have to pay, then online banking can make it a cakewalk because they can be paid automatically. If you are not so savvy with computers and that is what is pushing you back from online banking, don't worry, it's not that tough. But in any case, you can always ask a family member or a friend for help.

Sort through your credit cards and see what you need and what you don't. The more cards you have, the more you will get confused. So, it is always better to stick only a few cards that will give you more benefits than the others. If companies are bothering you with new card offers, read the terms very carefully and then judge whether you truly need them or your current card is enough to cover everything.

Always have a few hundred dollars in your apartment in someplace safe. This will serve as a backup in case the ATMs are closed, or there is a power outrage. If you keep misplacing your wallet every day before leaving the house, try using a wallet that is colorful. When your wallet is black or brown in color, they tend to mix with other things, and you cannot spot them at once. But when it has a bright color, it becomes easier to spot them.

Prioritize Your Happiness and Health

Most people don't realize how important it is to put their health before everything else. No matter where you are, you should always have some extra ADHD medication at hand. Whenever you are writing things in your planner, make sure you check your medication and note down the date when you need to refill it. In this way, you will never run out of medication.

You can even set a reminder alert on your phone to remind you when you need to buy new meds. But the date you are setting for refilling your medication should be at least a week before you run out of meds.

Your schedule should not only be about work. You should keep ample space in your schedule for socializing. Taking care of yourself also means that you need to meet people and go out with them. If you are an avid reader, then join a book club. If you love fitness, join a yoga class. Do what you love but make time for yourself.

Another thing that really helps ADHD patients is joining ADHD support groups. These groups can do wonders to how you see your life. They provide a lot of emotional support on days when you don't feel like doing anything. Everything that you are going through, the group members have gone through as well. So, why not share your experiences? There are a lot of in-person and online groups that you can check out.

Make Decisions Within a Time Limit

Making decisions can be quite overwhelming for an ADHD patient, and the main reason behind this is that they end up being so confused that making a decision seems next to impossible. Some patients can even spend weeks agonizing over the same issue over and over again. However, when analyzed by someone else, those decisions should not take you more than a couple of minutes. If you are going through the same thing, then one of the simplest was to solve it is to set a time limit. When you have a time cap, you know that you have to make a decision by the end of that time cap. If you are deciding on which sofa you should buy, set a time cap and then make a resolution that you are going to make your final decision before your time cap is over.

Whenever you are making a decision, I know that there are a lot of factors and, thus, a lot of angles to think from. But you need not think about everything. You have to prioritize and think about only some of the factors which are most important to you. It can be practicality, price, aesthetics, or anything else. The factors should be chosen by their importance. Stick to one factor for your ultimate decision.

Don't Over-Commit

We all have a tendency to overcommit. But you have to hold yourself back from doing so. When people have ADHD, they have a hard time keeping track of everything in their life. So, when you over-commit, you have a lot of things on your plate, and you cannot possibly handle all of them. If you spread yourself too thin, none of the tasks can be completed properly. So, commit to one task at a time and don't take up too much work at a time. You have to prioritize your own mental health over anything else.

Your To-Do Lists Should Not Be Too Long

Making to-do lists is definitely a great way to start the day and keep track of all those things you need to do, but it is also very easy to get lost in them. So, it is my advice to you that you keep your to-do lists short. Your list should have the tasks written in bold and big letters and don't list more than five or six tasks on the list. If there any additional tasks, write them on the back of the index card, and you will do those tasks only if you have time left after completing the major ones. When you see that your list is becoming short and you don't have too many things on the same page, you will automatically feel less frustrated. This will make completing tasks much easier.

Limit Your Distractions

There are too many distractions in our everyday life, but there is a way to fight them. You simply have to take the first step. Organizing your life will become way too difficult if you don't steer clear of all the distractions. When you are working, your focus should be solely on your work. Put your phone in the silent mode, and don't look at it for the next fifteen minutes. You can check your email after that and then return back to work for another fifteen minutes. Free your workspace of any clutter. The more things you have on your desk, the more will be the distractions.

Lastly, I would say that you need to take it one project at a time. Once you have set your priority, focus on completing that before moving on to something else. This will ensure that before you start a new task, all the loose ends have been tied up. If you follow all these steps, you will gradually see that you are mastering the art of organization

Chapter VII

Conclusion

Conclusion

Thank you for making it through to the end of *ADHD Workbook for Adults*; let us hope that you were able to get answers to all the questions you had in mind. I hope you have gained some knowledge from the insight that I shared in this book. Each and every strategy that has been mentioned in this book has been proven to bring the symptoms of ADHD under control and make your life easier.

The next step is to apply these strategies in your life so that you can lead a more fulfilled life with your loved ones. I understand that it is not always easy to deal with the symptoms of ADHD every day. It takes a lot of courage to tackle your issues head-on and put in all the hard work that is required to overcome the problems. It is quite probable that the first medicate you take, or the first therapy you seek might not work for you. But don't let that one moment discourage you from the path of seeking treatment because the right treatment is out there; you simply have to find it. There might be several instances where you have to try medications that are not the right fit for you, but only after you try things you will come to know what works for you and what doesn't. I had personally known so many people who had had to try several therapies and medications before they finally got 'the one' they had been looking for. The idea is to never lose hope.

Every journey has its own setbacks, and yours is no different. But there is no need to beat yourself up for a couple of failures. You need to keep reminding yourself to stay strong. Love yourself and give yourself a pat on the back whenever you make the least progress. Tell yourself that every challenge that comes on your path is just another opportunity for you to grow as a human being and learn new things along the way.

The one advice that I give to everyone is that if you want success in your battle against ADHD, you first have to learn how to accept yourself. No matter how many failures you receive, you have to stay excited and motivated for the new opportunities to come. Whenever you are starting to walk on a new path, it is always better that you start with a note of positivity. A positive mind will take you places. Just because you have ADHD doesn't mean that you cannot have a balanced life. You simply have to learn how you can work together with other people and improve your communication skills. If things seem too much to handle on your own, learn to delegate because it is always better to take help from others than do a task all by yourself and ruin it.

You will notice that organization is not your strongest skill set, but you have to come up with something practical that you can follow in your life. Take help from your close people or your family members whom you trust. Think about how you can come up with a system of planning things that will be easier to memorize and not much of a hassle. The moment you come up with a routine, your life will seem less chaotic because now, you have a set of tasks to complete within certain time frames. You should even plan your sleep and your meals so that you don't forget anything.

Agreeing to do too many things at a time can cause a lot of trouble in your life. But your tendency to become impulsive will force you to indulge in such behaviors. That is why it is important for every ADHD patient to learn to say no. The more work you take, the more jam-packed your routine is going to become, leaving you stresses and overwhelmed. Your ability to lead a lifestyle that is healthy depends largely on how well you prioritize your work and other commitments. So, whenever someone presents you with a new opportunity, take a moment to check your schedule and see how much you already have on your plate.

Don't pay heed to any of the ADHD myths or rumors in your surroundings. If you want to know something about ADHD, always read articles from trustworthy pages. Don't let anyone make you feel that you are lazy or using ADHD as an excuse. ADHD is a very real problem, and it is a disorder. Choose your therapist wisely because he/she is going to help you a lot in managing your symptoms.

There are so many challenges that ADHD patients have to face in their day-to-day life. From organizational difficulties to problems in time management, they have to put in more effort than others even when they are doing the simplest tasks. ADHD patients who already have a challenging job to handle find it even more difficult because it is no easy task. But take it one step at a time. Don't try to change everything all at once because that will only leave you even more overwhelmed. No matter what you do, don't overlook the stress that you are taking upon yourself. Keep a check on the stress levels. Engage in some physical activity even if it means going for a stroll in the neighborhood and eat a healthy diet. Practicing these healthy habits will also benefit you in the long-term by reducing your symptoms. Slowly, you will see how manageable your life becomes. Lastly, I would also encourage you to practice mindfulness and yoga, both of which will help in calming your mind. It will also help you exercise greater control over yourself and your emotions. If you are just a beginner, meditate for a shorter time span, and then you can gradually increase it.

I hope that the treatment options and the tips that I had mentioned in this book have come of help to you. If you doubt that you have been suffering from this disorder, then you should not be wasting any more time and meet the doctor at once. The longer you take to seek professional help, the more your condition will deteriorate. The right treatment is out there in front of you, and all you need to do is ask for it.

Finally, I would highly appreciate it if you can leave a review on Amazon if this book has helped you in any manner.

Chapter VIII

Resources

Resources

Alexander T. Vazsonyi, J. M. (2017). It's time: A meta-analysis on the self-control-deviance link. *Journal of Criminal Justice, 48*, 48-63.

Amelia Villagomez, U. R. (2014). Iron, Magnesium, Vitamin D, and Zinc Deficiencies in Children Presenting with Symptoms of Attention-Deficit/Hyperactivity Disorder. *Children, 1*(3), 261-279.

Anne Halmøy, O. B. (2009). Occupational Outcome in Adult ADHD: Impact of Symptom Profile, Comorbid Psychiatric Problems, and Treatment. *Journal of Attention Disorders, 13*(2), 175-187.

Aparajita B. Kuriyan, W. E. (2012). Young Adult Educational and Vocational Outcomes of Children Diagnosed with ADHD. *Journal of Abnormal Child Psychology, 41*(1), 27-41.

Benjamín Piñeiro-Dieguez, V. B.-M.-G.-L. (2016). Psychiatric Comorbidity at the Time of Diagnosis in

Adults With ADHD. *Journal of Attention Disorders, 20*(12), 1066-1075.

Joel T. Nigg, K. L. (2012). Meta-Analysis of Attention-Deficit/Hyperactivity Disorder or Attention-Deficit/Hyperactivity Disorder Symptoms, Restriction Diet, and Synthetic Food Color Additives. *Journal of the American Academy of Child & Adolescent Psychiatry, 51*(1), 86-97.

John T. Mitchell, L. Z. (2015). Mindfulness Meditation Training for Attention-Deficit/Hyperactivity Disorder in Adulthood: Current Empirical Support, Treatment Overview, and Future Directions. *Cognitive and Behavioral Practice, 22*(2), 172-191.

1. Eugene Arnold, N. L. (2012). Artificial Food Colors and Attention-Deficit/Hyperactivity Symptoms: Conclusions to Dye for. *Neurotherapeutics, 9*(3), 599-609.

Michael H. Bloch, J. M. (2014). Nutritional Supplements for the Treatment of ADHD. *Child and Adolescent Psychiatric Clinics of North America, 23*(4), 883-897.

Rucklidge, J. J. (2010). Gender Differences in Attention-Deficit/Hyperactivity Disorder. *Psychiatric Clinics of North America, 33*(2), 357-373.

Saskia van der Oord, S. M. (2011). The Effectiveness of Mindfulness Training for Children with ADHD and Mindful Parenting for their Parents. *Journal of Child and Family Studies, 21*(1), 139-147.

Stéphanie Baggio, A. F. (2018). Prevalence of Attention Deficit Hyperactivity Disorder in Detention Settings: A Systematic Review and Meta-Analysis. *Frontiers in Psychiatry, 9.*

Stephen P. Hinshaw, E. B.-N. (2012). Prospective follow-up of girls with attention-deficit/hyperactivity disorder into early adulthood: Continuing impairment includes elevated risk for suicide attempts and self-injury. *Journal of Consulting and Clinical Psychology, 80*(6), 1041-1051.

Winston Chung, S.-F. J. (2019). Trends in the Prevalence and Incidence of Attention-Deficit/Hyperactivity Disorder Among Adults and Children of Different Racial and Ethnic Groups. *JAMA Network Open, 2*(11).

Ylva Ginsberg, J. Q. (2014). Underdiagnosis of Attention-Deficit/Hyperactivity Disorder in Adult Patients. *The Primary Care Companion For CNS Disorders.*

Zheng Chang, P. D. (2017). Association Between Medication Use for Attention-Deficit/Hyperactivity Disorder and Risk of Motor Vehicle Crashes. *JAMA Psychiatry, 74*(6), 597.

CPSIA information can be obtained
at www.ICGtesting.com
Printed in the USA
BVHW041541010621
608548BV00008B/2256